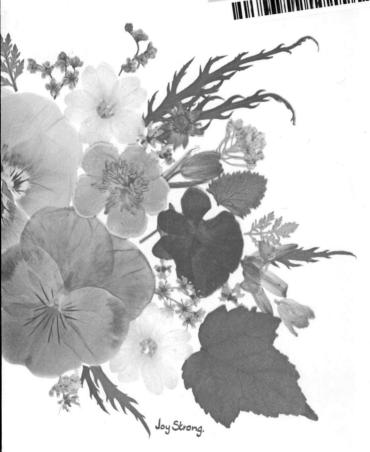

Joy Strong.

Pressed Flowers & Pot-pourri

A collection of traditional and original ideas for these most rewarding pastimes.

In the same series
NATURAL BISCUITS
NATURAL PÂTÉS
NATURAL SPICES

By the same author
A VEGETARIAN IN THE FAMILY
THE HOLISTIC COOK
ITALIAN DISHES
PASTA DISHES
PÂTÉS AND DIPS
PIZZAS AND PANCAKES
QUICHES AND FLANS
SIMPLE AND SPEEDY WHOLEFOOD COOKING
SNACKS AND STARTERS
THE RAW FOOD WAY TO HEALTH
THE WHOLEFOOD LUNCH BOX
THE WHOLEFOOD SWEETS BOOK

Edited by the author
THE VERY BEST OF VEGETARIAN COOKING

Pressed Flowers & Pot-pourri

by

David Eno

Illustrated by Joy Strong

THORSONS PUBLISHERS LIMITED
Wellingborough, Northamptonshire

Second revised edition published 1983
Second Impression 1984
Third Impression 1985

© THORSONS PUBLISHERS 1984

British Library Cataloguing in Publication Data

Eno, David
    Pressed flowers and pot-pourri.
    1. Flowers—Collection and preservation
    2. Perfumes   3. Flowers—Drying
    I. Title
    745.92   SB447

    ISBN 0-7225-0862-X

Printed and bound in Great Britain

CONTENTS

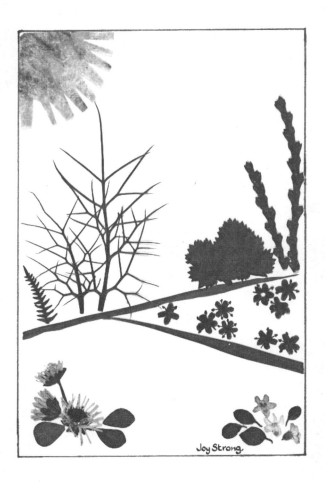

Joy Strong.

INTRODUCTION

The aim of this book is to provide sufficient information to give an understanding of the principles behind the pressing of flowers and the making of pot-pourri so that you can make best use of the particular materials available to you. You can create your own designs and evolve new recipes quite unique to your garden and personality. You could even go on to assemble a permanent botanical collection of favourite specimens, to treasure forever.

The processes involved are extremely simple and little equipment is needed to produce individual and charming results.

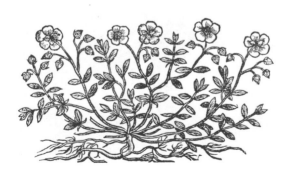

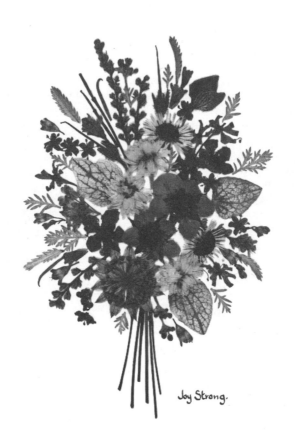

Joy Strong.

PART ONE:
PRESSED FLOWERS

THE FLOWER PRESS

I have successfully pressed flowers under heavy books, carpets, mattresses, boards weighted with bricks and even car seats when travelling. For consistent results however some type of press is desirable. One type is stocked by toy, gift and craft shops. This consists of two plywood squares held together by four bolts and wing nuts at the corners. Plants are pressed in sheets of blotting paper separated by corrugated card and the pressure can be adjusted by means of the wing nuts.

For those interested in doing a great deal of flower pressing a larger press would be desirable. A professional botanist's press, which is basically an arrangement of two stiff wire mesh rectangles kept under tension by small chains and springs, works very well. This has the advantage that it is large enough to cope with most plants and that the open mesh allows for rapid drying. Other suitable alternatives include book binding presses, trouser presses etc.

Other requirements are a pair of scissors, a pair of tweezers for arranging small delicate parts, a

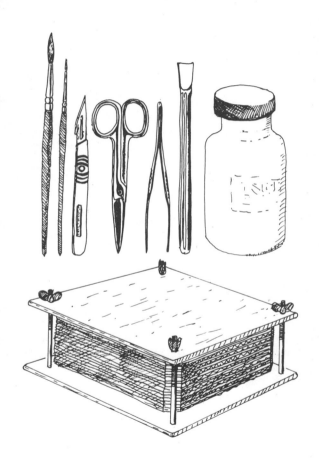

sharp knife or scalpel for thinning down bulky flowers and stems, a glue applicator and a small paint brush for applying small amounts of glue.

Materials

Although newsprint can be used for pressing, blotting paper is cleaner and more absorbent. White is best and cheapest if bought in large sheets from stationers. It can be used over and over again and is well worth the outlay.

Various glues can be used, although I have found, the P.V.A. type, such as 'Unibond' or 'Marvin Medium' to be particularly suitable. This type of glue is clean in use, virtually odourless and once dry becomes colourless and waterproof. One further advantage is that it may be thinned down with water and applied with a paint brush to small delicate stems and flowers.

In order to achieve any degree of permanence, pressed flowers should be mounted in such a way that they can he hermetically sealed. This may involve the use of transparent sticky film, which can be obtained from stationers, or varnish, or some kind of frame which must have a closely fitting back and glass. Secondhand frames can often be got cheaply from junk shops or jumble sales.

The only other requirement is a supply of paper, card or objects for mounting your flowers upon. This could include candles, paperweights, tablemats, book covers, door fingerplates, pebbles, trays, etc.

COLLECTING FLOWERS

Firstly a word about wild plants; many species are becoming scarce, and all over the world a number of plants become extinct each year. This is due almost entirely to the damaging effects of man's activities upon the environment.

The use of herbicides and the uprooting of hedges in intensive farming; the ever increasing development of roads; housing and industry; domestic and industrial pollution; these are among the things which have done and are doing irreparable damage to our environment. It is up to everyone to help preserve our heritage of flora and fauna, and therefore, before gathering wild plants, be absolutely sure they are growing in abundance. If uncertain then leave alone, or better still use only garden flowers, many of which, make excellent subjects for the flower press.

When collecting, choose undamaged flowers, and leaves, and pick when it is dry and sunny. If wet with dew or rain they will tend to go mouldy in the press. Always pick more material than you think you need as flowers can fall to pieces or get damaged during pressing, leaves may get bent or be of the wrong size for your intended purpose. In general try to select from each plant a representative sample of all its different parts, buds, flowers, seed heads, all the different-sized leaves, and, for those with a botanical interest, the roots too should be dug up and washed clean.

Do not be deterred from considering plants which are fleshy or succulent, or those which have large bulky flowers. While the plant as a whole may not be suitable for pressing, petals and leaves may be removed and pressed separately to be reassembled later. Stems can often be sliced in half to reduce thickness.

If you are collecting while out walking, certain plants may suffer from wilting before you reach home. Some kind of container will minimize this, a plastic bag is simple and effective but, to avoid crushing, a plastic sandwich box containing a layer of slightly damp cotton wool is even better.

If you are collecting for a botanical record it is usual to note the name of the plant, the habitat and any relevant details, e.g., sand dune, beech woodland, open meadow etc., the exact location, the date, and the name of the collector.

While searching for plants to press do not restrict yourself to flowering plants, as grasses, ferns, mosses and even seaweeds and some lichens can be used.

Lastly, remember not to be attracted only by large showy flowers but to consider all those small and possibly even miniscule plants which go unnoticed in their normal setting. When pressed and mounted they may be ideal for filling small spaces or for miniatures.

COLOUR

Colour Permanence

Most pressed and dried plants undergo some colour changes, and it is as well to have these in mind when you are selecting flowers. Much depends of course on the conditions under which they are pressed and stored, but more of this later.

As a very general rule many white, yellow, orange and pale flowers, keep their colours, while dark red, violet, blue and purple fade or change to grey and browns.

Green leaves change colour fairly rapidly, either fading to light grey-green, or in some cases turning almost black. Grey leaves, where the greyness is due to small hairs on the leaf, remain unchanged, and the same applies to silvery leaves.

The following table lists some useful plants for pressing and gives details of the changes which may be expected as they dry.

These changes however should not deter you as some of the resulting effects are quite beautiful.

As already suggested, the information given in the table is not absolute and depends upon many variable conditions. However, by understanding the reason for breakdown and discolouration of plant material it is at least possible to take some measures which will reduce this.

Mildew, discoloration and, to some extent,

fading are due to the action of fungi and bacteria which find the various chemical compounds within the plant a useful source of nutrition. Attack by these organisms, which are present everywhere, in the air, in dust, and on the surface of the plant, begins very soon after picking, although it may be some time before this becomes apparent.

Apart from food the one vital requirement for the growth of these organisms of decay is moisture. During pressing this is provided by the plant but if drying is sufficiently rapid they do not get a chance to gain a foothold.

Rapid drying is therefore essential to good preservation and may be achieved by the following methods. Firstly, thick pads of absorbent paper should be used during the first few days of pressing and these must be changed at least daily. Thick blotting paper is most suitable for this purpose and to avoid unnecessary disturbance of the plant while changing the pads it should be kept in a folder of thin, porous material. Thin paper will do if unsized, but better still is the non-woven fabric sold as interlining under the trade name 'Vilene'.

The blotting paper pads can be dried and re-used almost indefinitely, and, when the plant is dry, so can the folded retainers.

Secondly, drying can be speeded up by keeping the press in a warm dry place. An airing cupboard is ideal, but beware of too much heat as this can dry

A suggested list of suitable material to press:

Common Name	Botanical Name	Part Used*	Colour Change
Bells of Ireland	Molucella Laevis	F	—
Bluebell	Endymion Sp.	F	Blue to Creamy Beige
Bracken	Pteridium Aquilinium	L	Press at various stages for different colours
Broom	Cytisus Sp.	F	—
Bryony	Bryonia Dioica	L,F,T	—
Buttercup	Ranunculus Sp.	L,F,	Yellow-White over 3 years
Celandine	Ranunculus Ficaria	L,F,	Yellow-White over 1 year
Chives	Allium Schoenoprasum	L,F,	—
Clary	Salvia Sclarea	B	—
Clover	Trifoilum Sp.	F,L	—
Columbine	Aquilegia Sp.	F,L	—
Cuckoo Flower	Cardamine Pratensis	F,L	—
Daisy	Bellis Perennis	F,L,	—
Dog Rose	Rosa Canina	F,L	Cream-Brown
Elder	Sambucus Nigra	F	Beige
Forget-Me-Not	Myosotis Sp.	F,L	—
Foxglove	Digitalis Purpurea	F	Pink-Mauve
Golden Rod	Solidago Sp.	F	—
Gorse	Ulex Europaeus	F	Tan
Ground Ivy	Glechoma Hederacea	L	Purplish Leaf
Harebell	Campanula Sp.	F,L	All colour lost beautiful fragile white
Hawthorn, May	Crataegus Sp.	F,L	Beige to Cream
Heartsease	Viola Tricolor	F,L	Rapid change to shades of brown
Heath & Heather	Erica Sp.	F,L	Pick young stems
Hedge Parsley	Torilis	F,L	—
Herb Robert	Geranium Robertianum	L	Maroon leaves can be found
Honesty	Lunaria Annua	Seed Pod	Silver Inner Pod
Honeysuckle	Lonicera Sp.	F,L	Creamy Brown
Ivy	Hedera Helix	L	Green-Black

Common name	Botanical name	Parts	Notes
Jasmine-Yellow	Jasminum Sp.	F,L	Soft Beige
Jonquil	Narcissus Jonquilla	F,L	—
Lady's Mantle	Alchemilla Mollis	F	—
Larkspur	Delphinium Sp.	F	—
Lily of the Valley	Convallaria Majalis	F	Rapid change from Blue
Love-in-a-Mist	Nigella Damascena	F,L	Delicate Mauve
Mallow	Malva Sp.	F	Wide range of autumn colours
Maple	Acer Sp.	L	Yellow to transparent Beige in 1 year approx.
Marsh Marigold	Caltha Palustris	F	—
Meadowsweet	Filipendula Ulmarta	F	Good Creamy colour heavy pressing needed
Moon Daisy	Chrysanthemum Leucanthemum		—
Nipplewort	Lapsana Communis	Buds & F	Deep Maroon to Dark Brown
Peaony	Paeonia Sp.	Petals	—
Pampas Grass	Cortaderia Sp	Seeds	Blue & Violet change rapidly to Browns & Dark shades
Pansy	Viola Sp.	F	
Poppy-Red	Papaver Sp.	F	Soft shades of Pink
Polyanthus	Primula Vulgaris	F	Red presses Black
Primrose	Primula Vulgaris	F	Shades of Yellow & Lime Green
Rosebay Willowherb	Epilobium Angustifolium	F,L	—
Sage	Salvia Officianlis	F,L	—
Salvia	Salvia Horminum	B	—
Snowdrop	Galanthus Sp.	F	—
Tamarisk	Tamarix Anglica	—	,
Thrift	Armeria Maritima	F,L	—
Thyme	Thymus Sp.	F,L	—
Vetch	Vicia Sp.	F,T	—
Violet	Viola	F	Soft Violet to Brown
Wallflower	Cherianthus Sp.	F	—

*Key to parts used — F Flower, L Leaf, B Bract

Acknowledgement: The information in the above table was kindly supplied by Joy Strong.

to the point of brittleness and makes plants difficult to handle.

Thirdly, fresh plants should not be stacked up in the press in large numbers, and should be kept well separated from plants which are already partially dried. Sheets of thick card are best used as dividers and will to some extent limit the spread of dampness.

Colour permanence after pressing

After mounting, flowers should be sealed in some way to prevent dampness and insects from attacking. Sunlight is detrimental to nearly all floral pigments, and even bright indirect light causes fading. The final resting place for pictures or ornaments using pressed flowers should therefore be chosen.

Leaving plants for a year or so after pressing, as recommended later, allows colour changes to take place before use and helps avoid disappointment.

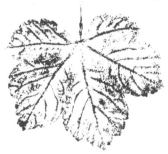

PRESSING

Having assembled your flower press, blotting paper, folders, card, and a selection of flowers and leaves of approximately equal thickness, arrange them in one of your blotting paper or Vilene folders. Remove any particulalry thick parts with a scalpel or pair of scissors. Try to persuade any unruly leaves or petals to remain flat by gentle pressing with your fingers. Any particularly difficult plants will have to be given a folder to themselves for the first day until they become more easy to manage.

Avoid folding petals or leaves as this generally leaves a permanent crease mark. After pressing for a day or two further arrangement is often easy and each folder should be checked anyway. Use thick pads of blotting paper for the first few days and change them daily putting them in a warm place to dry out. Use fairly gentle pressure for the first day or so, as too heavy a pressure will squeeze out the sap, distorting the plant and staining the flowers. Gentle initial pressure will also allow for freer air movement and more rapid drying. Gradually increase pressure as drying continues, and this will allow any short term colour changes to take place, and will avoid disappointment later. Indeed if you intend to go into pressed flower work in a serious way it is best to think a year or so ahead and lay in reasonably large stocks to cope with your future needs.

19

Seaweeds and Pondweeds

The more delicate seaweeds and pondweeds need a slightly different technique. They should be floated in a shallow dish of fresh water, allowing them a few minutes to fan themselves out into a natural position. A sheet of paper is then slid underneath and gently lifted out carrying with it the weed. Allow any surplus water to drain off, then leave on a flat surface for an hour or so. While still damp, place in a folder and press gently. Increase the pressure a little each day until completely dry.

The end result of this is that the weed becomes firmly attached to the paper, and no further attention is required. Other types of pressed materials can of course be added.

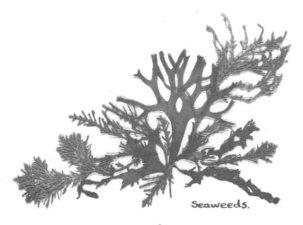

Seaweeds.

LAYOUT AND MOUNTING

Layout, design, and uses of pressed flowers

There are many ways of using pressed flowers, from framed pictures, both large and miniature, to cards, calendars, book marks, paperweights, candles, boxes, trays, tablemats, fingerplates, writing paper and many more.

Good design in the way your flowers are used and laid out is of the utmost importance, but unfortunately this is no easy matter to explain in a few lines, nor is it something which can be instantly appreciated. Effective design comes mainly from practice, but also from observing the work of others.

A single pansy mounted alone makes a beautiful picture and a satisfying result for the beginner.

However no-one can afford to be satisfied with their results for too long, and the more quickly you begin to find fault with your last piece of work the more quickly you are learning. Although it is easy to appreciate good design it is much more difficult to be able to pinpoint why you like it or indeed to produce a good design yourself. Trial and error will help you improve and a friend or teacher may be able to point out your mistakes more quickly than you can see them yourself.

So far I have given little practical advice, so here are a few points which will help start you in the right direction. Begin with simple arrangements using only a few flowers and leaves. Many people find it easier to work on a small scale and leave larger compositions until they have built up confidence. Try to make one focal point of interest, this could be a single flower or a group of flowers. The rest of the composition should lead the eye to this point by being subordinate to it. A composition with a number of competing focal points is confusing and not pleasing.

Always consider your design with respect to the space it is to occupy. If, for instance, you are making a six inch frame don't do it on a larger piece and cut it down afterwards. Start with the right size and shape of paper or card for the job you are doing.

As regards colour, which is a whole subject in itself, it is difficult to do wrong with pressed flowers as they take on a mellow colouration which makes them blend well. A coloured background, if not overpowering, can often improve a composition or help your inspirational powers. A composition which is turning out to be rather drab can often be helped by some small areas of intense colour. Try not to use too many different colours, but stick to a colour theme, shades of one colour, perhaps with a little of the complementary to give a lift, or autumn or spring colours. There are many different approaches and absolutely no fixed rules.

Another aspect of your composition is the subject matter. Many will be quite content to let the flowers themselves be the subject and confine themselves to achieving pleasing arrangements. However you may wish to depict other subjects such as birds, butterflies or other animals, or even landscapes.

Mounting

The points which follow apply generally to mounting for whatever application. A later section deals with the problems associated with specific applications.

There are two methods of working. For beginners it is best to lay out all the flowers, moving them around until you achieve a satsifactory arrangement, and then glue afterwards. For the more experienced each part can be glued down as you go, although obviously this leaves no room for error.

All pressed material is prone to curling, and so a mixture of thin and thick flowers in one picture will inevitably leave gaps which will allow the thinner parts to distort, therefore use only flowers of the same thickness for a particular piece of work. If the work is to be covered with adhesive film use only very thin plants to avoid unsightly air pockets, spoiling the results.

Although stiff paper can be used as a base to work on thin card is better and is available in a range of colours at most stationers and art shops.

Use the absolute minimum of glue applied in small spots to the plants themselves. A matchstick or a piece of very thin dowelling is a good tool to use for applying the glue. Large blobs of glue will spread and make a mess and soak into the plant leaving unsightly stains. The P.V.A. glue already mentioned sticks rapidly and any parts which will not stay flat need only be held down for a minute or two. Keeping your plants under pressure until needed and also working on a flat surface will reduce the need for this.

All finished or partly finished work should be stored in a press or under some heavy books until it can be framed or finished.

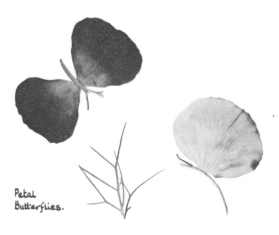

Petal
Butterflies.

PICTURES

Make sure when working that vital parts of the design are not cut off by the edges of the frame. Although you may wish to leave the consideration of the frame until last it will be cheaper and save much trouble if you obtain a secondhand or new ready-made frame and work to this.

Although you may fill the frame completely with your picture, a more professional-looking result is obtained by mounting the picture onto a larger sheet of contrasting colour. Window-type mounts should not be used as these leave a gap which will allow crinkling and distortion.

In addition to the picture and the sheet of stiff strawboard, mounting board, or preferably hardboard, is needed for a backing. The picture can be sealed between the glass and the hardboard before placing in the frame by using gummed paper tape or special book repairing tape around the edges. Ordinary Sellotape comes unstuck.

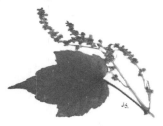

PAPERWEIGHTS AND OTHER PRESENTS

Paperweights

Having obtained a plain glass paperweight, cut a circle of thin card or paper which is very slightly smaller than the flat part of the base. Onto this circle of paper stick your pressed flowers. The easiest type of design starts off with a central flower and builds around this, although asymmetrical designs can be just as effective if done carefully. It is best to choose thin, uniform material so that the paperweight will rest flat when finished.

The base is finished with a circle of felt or leather cut slightly larger than the paper circle. The design is stuck onto the felt circle with a small amount of glue, and this should leave a small margin of felt showing. A strong clear glue such as 'Durofix' should then be spread thinly along this margin and the paperweight lowered carefully into position.

Candles

The addition of pressed flowers to candles is quick and easy. The candle should be left in a warm place until the wax begins to soften. Flowers and leaves can now be carefully pressed into the soft surface of the candle. Once you have completed the design the candle can be dipped into molten wax and hung up by its wick to cool.

Greetings cards, gift tags, bookmarks

Greetings cards, gift tags, bookmarks and many other stationary items can be made with pressed flowers, Once the pressed flowers are glued down, a sheet of transparent sticky film is applied, such as that sold for covering books. The sheet of film should be cut somewhat larger than the work to be covered and trimmed down later. The application of the film can be quite tricky especially over large areas. The best method is to peel only one corner of film off its backing paper with one hand, with the other you rub down the adhesive film. If done carefully this should avoid unsightly air bubbles being trapped.

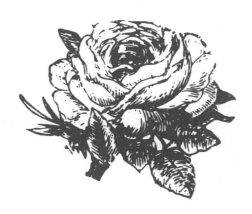

PART TWO:
POT-POURRI

THE BACKGROUND TO
POT-POURRI

In this section the emphasis is on using plants which can be grown in an English garden. Almost every garden contains at least a few plants which can provide suitable material and should you wish to obtain more I have included a list of suppliers at the back of the book. Some of the plants required such as roses, lavender, sweet peas, violets, carnations and lily of the valley are part of the mainstay of the traditional flower garden. Other useful plants are found among the culinary and medicinal herbs. Most of these are easy to cultivate, tolerant of a variety of soil conditions, and make attractive additions to the garden. Quite apart from avoiding the expense of buying ready-prepared ingredients it is so much more satisfying to see the process through from beginning to end. If you are unable to grow any of the ingredients they can be obtained ready-dried and prepared from various sources and these I also list at the back of the book.

Many commercial and old time recipes include ingredients which do not originate from temperate climes and in places I give suggestions for the use of these. While they do increase the range of possibilities they are by no means essential. The only ingredients which you cannot grow yourself that are very useful are spices such as cloves, cinnamon, allspice, nutmeg etc., but these are easy enough to obtain.

The use of fragrant plants for scenting dwellings is of great antiquity. Not only were they used to drive away unpleasant smells in times when ventilation and sanitation were poor and houses damp, but also many curative properties were, and still are, attributed to them. The aromatic oils present in such plants as cinnamon, lavender rosemary and eucalyptus are known to have antibacterial properties and in the past plague was kept away by burning bundles of dried juniper, rue, lavender, bay and other aromatic plants.

Churches and other public meeting places had their floors strewn with sweet smelling herbs, and the burning of aromatics such as incense is an integral part of many religious ceremonies. These practices would seem to have had a highly practical aspect in the past when medicine was less well developed and fatal infectious diseases were more frequent.

The plants used for strewing on floors included mints, lavender, thyme, hyssop, tansy, rosemary, sage, sweet flag and balm. It was a natural development from this practice to begin the making of fragrant bowls for scenting rooms, and pomanders for wearing about the neck both to scent the body and keep it free from infection.

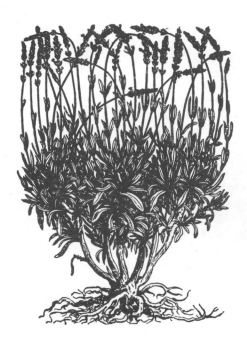

THE COMPOSITION OF
POT-POURRI

What goes into pot-pourri is very much a matter of personal preference and of what ingredients you have available; the range of possible ingredients is very large. However there are certain things which should be present in fairly fixed proportions and to simplify matters these can be divided into four categories as follows:

1. Predominant perfuming agent
2. Underlying perfumes
3. Fixatives
4. Preservatives.

The following sections deal with each of these in turn and at the end a general recipe is given suggesting quantities of each of these components.

PERFUMES

Predominant Perfume

Although roses traditionally predominate in pot-pourri on account of their remarkable and lasting fragrance, they can play a subordinate role or be dispensed with completely if you prefer a herbal mixture. Although any scented rose may be used those with the strongest scents are *rosea centifolia* (The Hundred Leaved Rose), *R. damascena* (The Damask Rose), *R. indica* (The Tea Rose), and the numerous hybrids derived from them.

Lavender plays an important part in traditional recipes and here again its popularity is due to its refreshing and lasting fragrance. It blends well with roses but should be used sparingly because of it's strength.

The following could be used either alone or in combination:

Flowers:

Pinks and Carnations, Lilac, Violet, Heliotrope, Jonquil, Orange, Grapefruit and Lemon, Jasmine, Meadowsweet, Wallflower, Magnolia, Magnolia, Nicotiana, Migionette, Mahonia, Arnica, Hyacinth Broom.

Leaves:

Woodruff, Melilot, Rosemary, Bergamot,

Costmary, Spearmint, Applemint, Gingermint,
Pineapple Mint, Eau de Cologne Mint,
Pennyroyal, Orange Mint, Sage, Pineapple Sage,
Santolina, Lemon Geranium, Rose Geranium,
Lemon Balm, Petaragonium, Basil, Lemon
Verbena, Southernwood, Sweet Briar, Bay
Laurel, Birch Buds, Clary Sage, Eucalyptus,
Camphor Plant, Calamint, Thyme, Lemon
Thyme.

Roots:
Angelica, Sweet Flag, Ginger.

Seeds:
Aniseed, Coriander, Fennel.

Your choice is governed only by what you like and
what you can grow. The selection above is by no
means exhaustive but most of the plants mentioned
have scents with a fair degree of permanence. You
will probably think of many other scented plants but
very often their perfume disappears completely
upon drying; however this is something which you
can determine by experiment.

Underlying perfumes
These can be supplied by a number of ingredients
which are added in smaller amounts so that they
subtly blend with the main body of the mixture.

There are a number of herbs which fall into this category, for example:

Thyme, Sweet Marjoram, Sage, Bay, Lavender, Santolina or Cotton Lavender, Tansy, Pelargonium, Rose Geranium, Lemon Geranium, Lemon Verbena, Peppermint, Lemon Balm, Lemon Thyme, Basil, Tarragon.

Spices can be added, such as:

Cinnamon, Nutmeg, Allspice, Ginger, Cardamom, Coriander, Anise, Fennel Seed.

These can be added either in ground or whole form; in the latter case the scent is given off more sparingly over a longer period.

The peel of lemons, oranges or limes is also a most useful ingredient giving a sharpness and freshness which is an improvement to most pot-pourri. The peel should be removed from a whole fruit either with sharp knife or coarse grater, so that the pith is left behind.

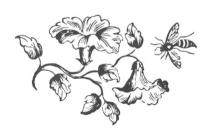

FIXATIVES

The Fixative

Although the recipes for pot-pourri, sachets, pomanders etc., can be varied entirely to your own taste and resources there is one ingredient which is essential and this is the fixative.

Plants owe their scents mainly to a variety of aromatic oils, waxes and resins which are produced in various parts of the plant. Some of these oils evaporate very slowly and consequently impart a lasting perfume, whilst others are extremely volatile and present only in minute quantities, for example the floral perfumes like Jasmine and Violet. The fixative helps to preserve these delicate and transient pefumes and although this action is not fully understood its is thought that the fixative, which is usually an oil or wax of low volatility, combines with the perfume oil and renders it less volatile. The fixative is often strongly scented iself and this must be taken into account when using it.

In commercial perfumery various fixatives of animal origin are employed such as musk, ambergris, civet and castor and these are sometimes cited in pot-pourri recipes. However there are plenty of alternatives of plant origin which do not entail the exploitation of animals. Perhaps the most useful and easiest to obtain is orris root which is not the root, but the rhizome of various irises. This has its own intense violet perfume and is used commercially as an ingredient in violet-scented compounds.

Orris Root
Orris Root comes from the thick, partly buried rhizomes of *Iris germanica, I. pallida* and *I. florentina* and their hybrids. These are very easily cultivated and are widely grown for their ornamental value. Before you decide to buy plants it might be as well to establish the identity of any irises you may already have in your garden, or alternatively you can test a piece of rhizome.

The best time for gathering the rhizomes is towards the end of summer and, to obtain the highest yield of the aromatic principle, it is best to prevent flowering on the sections of the plant which you intend to harvest. After harvesting, all the small rootlets should be removed and the surface skin peeled away. Don't be put off by an acrid smell which may be present initially. It is only after drying that the violet perfume develops, and continues to intensify for two years or more, due to chemical changes which take place within the rhizome. Thorough drying in a warm place is important and can be hastened by slicing or grating the rhizomes.

Although the scent is not identical to that of violets, Orris is the basis of many violet pefumes, toilet waters and extracts. Powdered Orris used to be added to the final rinsing water of linen and clothes and imparted a refreshing perfume. Beads and small ornaments can be carved or turned out of Orris Root and the scent lasts for years.

Other Fixatives

In commercial pefumery, a substance known as coumarin is used both as a fixative and to impart the scent of new mown hay. This substance is present in some grasses and is indeed responsible for the smell of hay. It is also found in more concentrated form in plants such as Melilot, Woodruff and Meadowsweet and these are frequent ingredients in pot-pourri recipes. The delightful scent is present only after drying.

Four species of Melilot (*melilotus sp.*) are found growing wild in this country. Although it was originally introduced as a fodder crop it has now been replaced by clover and lucerne. The bushy plants grow up to 4 feet high on roadsides, railway embankments and waste ground and have racemes of yellow or white papilionaceous flowers. The seeds are obtainable from suppliers and grow easily. For use in pot-pourri collect the whole plant while in flower and hang in bunches in a warm place to dry. When brittle chop into small pieces with scissors, and store in an airtight container. Incidentally Melilot is also an excellent bee plant.

Woodruff (*Galium ordoratum*) is a native of this

country and is farily common in woods and shady places and can be obtained from suppliers. The plant is gathered and dried whole as for Melilot.

Meadowsweet, also a common plant in moist places should be treated in the same way as Melilot.

Sweet Flag (*Acorus calamus*) is an introduced plant which is now fairly well distributed in the south of England. The whole plant is sweetly scented and was formerly used for strewing on the floors of churches, castles and houses. It is found growing with it's roots submerged in water and if you can get hold of a piece and you have a suitable wet patch in your garden it will grow rapidly. The root is the main part used and should be sliced and dried. For use as a fixative double the amount you would use for Orris, or use a mixture. The powdered root is known as Calamus powder.

Tonka or Tonquin Beans also contain coumarin and are imported from Brazil and Guyana and are fairly easy to obtain.

Gum Benzoin or Benjamin is also a useful fixative which comes from the resin exuded by Styrax Benzoin, a tree native to Thailand and Sumatra. You may be able to obtain this from a local chemist either as a tincture or in the resin form.

One note of caution; the wild plants of this country are already diminishing due to man's devastation of the countryside. Please do be conscientious and pick wild plants only sparingly and only if they are really abundant. If less than abundant do not disturb at all but obtain plants from a supplier. It requires an effort by everyone of us to preserve what is left of our countryside.

Lastly, the essential oils of Patchouli, Sandlewood and Vetivert are readily obtained from Indian shops and some chemists. These should be sprinkled very sparingly into your mixture one drop at a time until the desired effect is achieved as they have their own persistent scent.

The Preservative

The Preservative has no direct effect upon the perfume of the pot-pourri, but is responsible for preventing the decay of the constituent leaves, flowers and roots due to the action of micro-organisms and insects.

In older recipes Bay Salt was called for, this being a rather impure form of ordinary salt. Sea Salt is a satisfactory alternative, preferably as a mixture of coarse and fine grades. This should be dried in a very low oven for several hours before use. An alternative to salt is Borax, which is obtainable from chemists.

In all cases dryness is essential to ensure good keeping qualities and this can be aided by using small cotton bags of silica gel, about ½oz (15g) per container. This can be dried out occasionally by baking in a very low oven.

MAKING POT-POURRI

General Recipe for Pot-Pourri
1. Predominant perfume, 3 pints (1½ litres approx) of *dried* flowers or leaves.
2. Underlying perfumes, up to ¾ pint (½ litre approx) of dried flowers or leaves in any combination (but only ¼ pint of lavender flowers). In addition up to ¼ pint dried spice (or up to ½ pint for very spicy mixtures and the outer rind of 1-2 citrus fruits, grated.

   Essential oils, up to 3 drops of persistent types (Patchouli, Vetivert, Sandalwood) and up to 10 drops of milder types (Poppy, Imitation Musk, Lavender, Rosemary, Lemon, Frangipani etc.).
3. Fixatives, 1½ oz (45 grams) of Orris, double the quantity of any of the other of the fixatives mentioned.
4. Preservative, up to ½ pint.

Methods of making Pot-Pourri
There are two methods of making pot-pourri and each has its merits. The dry method entails complete drying of all the ingredients before they are mixed and better preserves the colour of the flowers.

The moist method results in better preservation of the scent but in the process the ingredients become discolored. This method is particularly applicable when rose petals are used. Whether the appearance of the finished product is important or not depends on what containers you intend to use. Most of the original containers were opaque ceramic bowls and consequently the appearance was of no concern.

The Dry Method

Absolute dryness of all ingredients is essential. In order to achieve this without too much loss of the volatile essential oils the ingredients should be gathered when the dew has lifted and should then be placed in a warm shady place where there is free air circulation. A temperature of about 70°F (21°C) is ideal. Petals and flowers should be spread upon trays or, better still, wooden frames with muslin or orangdie stretched across them. As a general rule flowers should be gathered just after they have opened. Larger flowers such as roses, lilies and magnolias should have their petals removed as it is these which carry the perfume. Smaller flowers such as lily of the valley, hyacinth and jasmine should be removed whole from their stems. Herbs should be hung to dry in bunches.

As soon as the ingredients are dry and crisp they should be mixed with some fixative and placed in airtight jars. Use about 1 oz (25g) of Orris root to 2 pints (1 litre) of dried petals, flowers or leaves. The various flowers and herbs can be stored in separate containers until you have the selection you require. In this way you can combine flowers from early

41

spring to late summer in your finished pot-pourri.

The final blending should be done in a large storage, or sweet jar and the flowers and herbs should be combined with the preservative and your selection of spices, citrus peel, essential oils etc. About 4 oz (100g) of silica gel in a cotton bag should also be added to ensure complete dryness. The jar should then be sealed and left to mature for about six weeks. After this time the pot-pourri can be put in containers for use.

The Moist Method

The petals are gathered and spread out to dry as before, but in this case they are only allowed to partially dry until of a leathery texture. This takes about 48 hours and in the process the petals loose one third to one half of their original volume. They are now placed in a large jar — a sweet jar is excellent — together with the sea salt mixture already described. Make a ½ inch (1cm) layer of petals and then sprinkle over a little salt and repeat until the jar is about two-thirds full. You should allow one cup of salt to two of petals and keep each new layer well pressed down. The jar can be filled over a period of a few days and this puts less strain on your flower garden, but stir the contents of the jar before adding fresh layers. Keep the jar tightly closed and in a dark place for about ten days. After this time your should find that the petals have formed a solid mass which should be removed and broken into pieces. These can now be added to the other ingredients in another large jar as in the dry method and allowed to mature for 6 weeks.

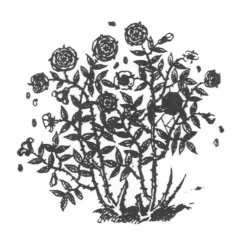

Containers for Pot-Pourri

All containers used for pot-pourri should have completely airtight lids. If pot-pourri were left exposed to the air continuously it would soon loose its perfume and also one would become so accustomed to it that one would not notice it. Jars and bowls with perforated lids only are not suitable, the original jars often had an outer airtight lid with an inner perforated lid.

Pot-pourri made by the dry method has an attractive appearance and this can be enhanced by adding dry rosebuds and other flowers for the sake of their appearance alone. This type of pot-pourri should be displayed in a glass container and there are many attractive storage jars on the market which are suitable. These can be found in chemists, hardware stores, kitchen shops and department stores and in antique and secondhand shops.

POMANDERS AND PASTILLES

The traditional pomander could be described as a concentrated pot-pourri compounded with gum or wax and rolled into a ball. This ball was often, although not always, enclosed in a decorative spherical container with perforations to let out the perfume. It was worn on a chain about the neck or waist where it perfumed the body, and helped ward off infection. More recently the container itself has come to be known as a pomander, but tracing the name to its French derivation *pomme d'ambre*, apple of ambergris, it clearly refers to the contents; ambergris being the name of the fixative derived from the whole which was commonly used as an ingredient.

The containers were often of precious metals, rare woods, or ivory intricately worked and are now highly prized as antiques. Modern containers are usually of china or porcelain and are often filled with pot-pourri. This is not particularly satisfactory because as I have already said pot-pourri tends to loose its perfume when constantly exposed to the air as it is in a pomander. The gum or wax in the traditional type helped fix the perfume there-by delaying its release and so I would recommend going to the extra trouble of making this type.

The ingredients and the quantities involved are extremely variable in old recipes and many ingredients are now difficult to obtain. However good results can quite easily be obtained by using a strongly scented pot-pourri mixture. To achieve this add a few drops of essential oil lavender, rosemary, vetivert etc., to a normal pot-pourri mixture. The best gum to use is gum tragacanth. This is usually in powder form and should be sprinkled a little at a time onto the surface of some water in a cup while stirring continuously. Keep adding until a thick consistency is achieved. Now stir enough of the gum into the pot-pourri to bind it into a solid mass. Roll this into balls and allow to dry and harden in a warm place. Gum tragacanth is expensive and possibly a cheaper gum such as acacia could be used, although I have not tried this.

As an alternative to gum, beeswax is very suitable and adds its own distinctive perfume. This should be melted and poured into the pot-pourri and the mixture quickly formed into balls. The finished pomanders can be drilled and hung on strings or ribbons. They may be hung inside clothes in a wardrobe or put in drawers or of course hung around the neck.

The word pomander is also used to refer to an orange stuck with cloves. This used to be made as a cheap alternative to real pomanders in poorer households although to my mind it is in no way inferior. Thin skinned oranges, limes or lemons can be used and the job is made easier by first puncturing the holes with a knitting needle. It is best to start from one end of the fruit and work in a spiral fashion, trying to space as evenly as possible while leaving a small gap between each clove. As the orange dries out the gaps will close up and any irregularity in spacing will tend to disappear. The pungent oil of cloves keeps away all fungi and bacteria and thus prevents decay of the orange. Eventually the orange dries completely and becomes very hard.

Immediately after sticking in the cloves you can sprinkle the orange with powdered nutmeg or cinnamon which adds to the delightful perfume.

Clove oranges make delightful presents and their appearance can be enhanced by tying a ribbon around them and packing in pot-pourri in a box. This type of pomander makes a good table decoration or can be used for scenting clothes and incidentally keeps away moths.

Pastilles or scented beads are really a variation of pomanders and are made with gum in exactly the same way. When hard they are drilled and threaded to make a scented necklace. The beads can be finished by turning on a lathe which gives them an attractive polished finish. Wax is not recommended for scented beads as the warmth of the body tends to soften it and it would soon rub away.

PILLOWS AND SACHETS

Herb Pillows

These are a continuation of the ancient tradition of stuffing mattresses with sweet herbs which was practised at least as far back as Roman times. The gentle aroma helps to soothe mind and body and to induce sleep. While the aroma of many plants may have a mild sleep inducing effect, hops are an age old remedy for insomnia and are definitely known to contain a volatile oil, which is sedative and soporific. Many other plants owe at least some of their effectiveness to their decongestant and anaesthetic action which is due to the substances such as camphor, menthol, thymol, and evgenol.

Particularly recommended are Thyme, Chamomile, Mints, Rosemary, Pine needles, Lemon Verbena, Lemon Balm, Lavender and Scented Geraniums.

Sachets and Sweet Bags

Sachets and sweet bags are used to scent clothing and may also be used to keep moths away if the right filling is employed. They are simply cloth bags filled with any aromatic material. Although the most well known filling is lavender many other fillings can be used either alone or in conjunction. Here are a few suggestions:

Orris Root, Melilot, Tonka Beans, Meadowsweet, Vetivert (leaves), Mint, Geranium, Lemon Balm, Bay Laurel, Calamus Powder, Basil, Thyme, Rose Petals, Sage, Camphor Plant, Eucalyptus, Bergamot, Southernwood, Calamint. In addition pot-pourri may be used as a filling.

For moth bags use a combination of some of all of the following fixed with Orris Root:

Rosemary, Rue, Southernwood Santolina, Camphor Plant, Thyme, Mint, Cloves, Lavender, Tansy, Wormwood and Melilot. Use in this case equal proportions of mixed herbs and Orris Root.

Suppliers of Plants, Seeds and Dried ingredients for Pot-Pourri.

The following is by no means a comprehensive list but I have tried to select growers who specialize in a useful selection of plants suitable for pot-pourri. Only some nurseries are open to the public, and many now charge for their descriptive catalogues, so in all cases send a stamped addressed envelope for information and always telephone before calling.

Suppliers of Plants and Seeds

ASHFIELDS HERB NURSERY, Hinstock, Market Drayton, Salop. Good general range of herb plants, including many suitable for pot-pourri. Seeds also stocked.

BETH CHATTO, White Barn House, Elmstead Market, Colchester, Essex. Catalogue entitled *Unusual Plants* is well worth buying. SAE for details.

CANDLESBY HERBS, Cross Keys Cottage, Candlesby, Spilsby, Lincs. Tel: Scremby 2111. Large selection of fresh herb plants. Herb garden open to visitors. Also fixatives, dried herbs essential oils, cosmetics etc. Telephone for details.

DORWEST HERB GROWERS, Bridport, Dorset. Free catalogue, good general selection of herb plants and seeds.

GREEN FARM COTTAGE HERBS, Thorpe Green, Thorpe Morieux, Bury St. Edmunds, Suffolk. Good general list of herb plants, very attractive catalogue.

THE HERB GARDEN, Thunderbridge, Kirkburton, W. Yorkshire. A good general range of herb plants.

HILLIER NURSERIES (WINCHESTER) LTD., Ampfield House, Ampfield, Romsey, Hants. Extensive range of plants stocked, herbaceous, shrubs and trees including roses and herbs. A range of more popular plants is stocked at the Hillier Garden Centre, Romsey Road, Winchester, Hants. Write or phone for details of descriptive list and books.

HOLLINGTON NURSERIES LTD, Woolton Hill, Newbury, Berks. RG15 9XT. Tel: (0635) 253908. An extensive selection of herb plants, many especially suitable for pot-pourri. Comprehensive catalogue available. Nursery open to visitors. Send SAE for list and further details.

OAK COTTAGE HERB FARM, Nesscliffe,

Shropshire. An interesting range of herb plants. Also a selection of dried herbs, lavender, pot-pourri, herb pillows, sachets.

THE OLD RECTORY HERB GARDEN, Ightham, Kent. Extensive range of herb plants and seeds, also dried lavender, lemon verbena, pomandes, and pot-pourri.

STOKE LACY HERB FARM, Herefordshire. Good general range of herb plants, also interesting half day courses are run.

SUFFOLK HERBS, Sawyers Farm, Little Cornard, Sudbury, Suffolk. Extensive range of organically grown culinary medicinal and ornamental herb plants. Specialize in a wide range of lavenders and rosemary. Also sell an extensive range of seeds.

VALESWOOD HERB FARM, Little Ness, Shropshire. SAE. General range of herb plants and also dried herbs and flowers for pot-pourri.

THE WEALD HERBARY, Park Cottage, Frittenden, Cranbrook, Kent. A good range of herbs listing many plants useful for pot-pourri.

YEW TREE HERBS, Holt Street, Nonington, Nr. Dover, Kent. SAE. Interesting catalogue listing many plants useful for pot-pourri.

Suppliers of dried and ready prepared ingredients

BALDWINS, 173, Walworth Road, London SE17. Herbalists stocking essential oils, floral essences, fixatives, spices, and an enormous range of dried herbs: 01-703 5550. Probably the most extensive stockist of herbal supplies. N.B. No postal service, callers only.

CHATTELS, 53 Chalk Farm Road, London NW1 8AN. Tel: 01-267 0877. Specialize in dried flowers and ready-made pot-pourris. Extensive range of seeds, essential oils and ingredients.

CRANKS LTD., Marshall Street, London W.1. Stock a wide range of herbs and spices. Branches also at Dartington, Totnes, and Guildford.

CULPEPER LTD. Personal Shopping: 21, Bruton Street, London W.1. 9 Flask Walk, Hampstead, NW3. 14 Bridwell Alley, Norwich. 25 Lion Yard, Cambridge. 4 Market Street, Winchester. 33 High Street, Corking. 12D Mettinghouse Lane, Brighton. 28, Milsom Road, Bath. Mail order from Culpeper Ltd., Hadstock Road, Linton, Cambridge. Dried Herbs, both medicinal and culinary, dried flowers, spices, essential oils, and a large range of attractively packaged pot-pourri, pillows, sachets, pomanders. Herb plants sold from shops but not by post.

HOLLINGTON NURSERIES LTD, Woolton Hill, Newbury, Berks. RG15 9XT. Tel: (0635) 253908. Wide selection of specially packaged dried ingredients for pot-pourri, essential oils fixatives etc. Also ready-made pot-pourri and gifts. Comprehensive catalogue available. Nursery open to visitors. Send SAE for list and further details.

GERRARD HOUSE, 736 Christchurch Road, Boscombe, Bournemouth, Dorset. Postal service dealing mainly with medicinal herbs and extracts but also stock some pot-pourri ingredients. Free catalogue.

Supplier of pressed flower equipment

JOY STRONG, 16 Everlands, Cam, Dursley, Gloucestershire. Starter pack containing 1 picture frame, 1 glass paperweight, 3 bookmark mounts, 6 medium and 6 mini cards with envelopes. No flowers included. SAE for details.

INDEX

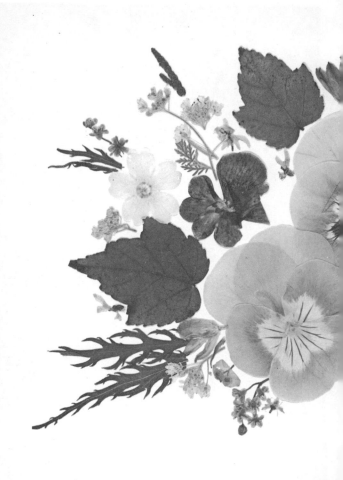